Pain Relief:

30 Homemade Remedies for With Essential Oils and Herbs

Table of Contents

Introduction

There you are, reading the back of another bottle, trying to find the relief you need. Your head hurts, your joints ache, and you just want to go home and feel better, but you don't want to take something that's going to throw you through a loop for the next few days.

You read the side effects and you read the ingredients. You don't know what half of them are, and you really don't know if that's what you should be putting in your body. When it comes to your health, you want to do what's best, not just to treat what you are feeling, but by what you put inside yourself, too.

Natural remedies are the only way to ensure you are doing what's right for your body without compromising the rest of your health. You can effectively treat what you want to treat, but you don't have to stress that by treating it you are going to expose yourself to a wealth of other symptoms.

But are natural remedies effective?

I want to try them, but I don't know how, and I don't know if they really work.

Modern medicine is better, isn't it? After all, it is modern.

If you have ever considered turning to natural remedies, odds are you have hesitations. But, with this book, I want to show exactly how to use essential oils and herbs effectively, getting the results you want without breaking the bank.

Let me show you the world of herbs and oils, and get you feeling back to your old self in no time.

You know you want to, so go for it. The natural way is the better way, always.

Chapter 1 – Herbal Remedies 101: An Overview

Long before modern medicine ever entered the scene, herbs have been used to treat a plethora of ailments. From headaches and body aches to joint pain and muscle cramps, you can find herbs to relieve all your symptoms, and get you back on your feet in no time.

However, not all herbs are the same, and it is important to know what you are using in your treatments. Though some herbs may taste better than others, or some herbs may sound more appealing than others, you have to know which ones work for which ailments before you try using them to treat yourself.

In this book, I want to show you how to use both herbs and essential oils in ways that you haven't before. I want to show you how you can use natural remedies to treat a variety of illnesses and health problems, and how you never need to step foot inside a doctor's office to do it.

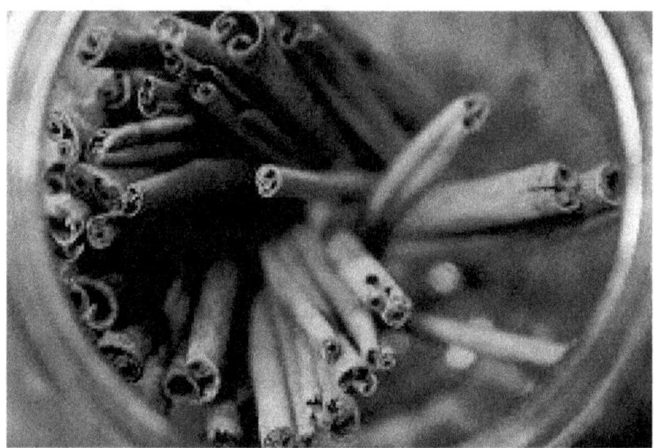

In this book, I want to show you how to use aromatherapy and teas to treat body aches and pains, and how you can use simple herbs around you to achieve the same health benefits expensive medication provides.

However, you are going to walk away better than ever knowing that you aren't faced with the same side effects you have to deal with when you use synthetic pills.

Though you must exercise moderation, you aren't going to have to monitor yourself for a list of symptoms when you take herbal remedies, because they are safe to use.

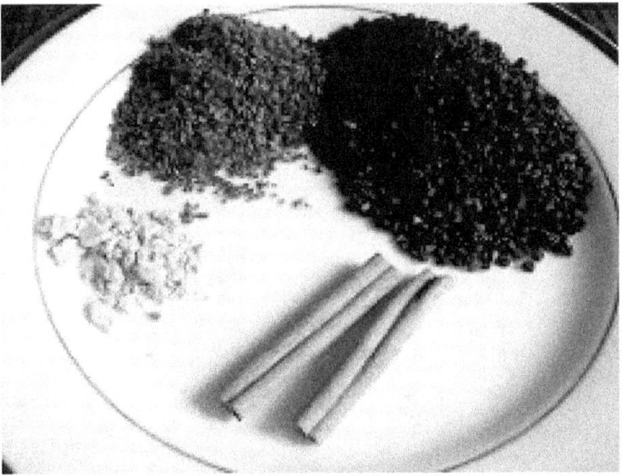

All you need to do is learn which herbs are right for the condition you are facing, then break up these dried herbs into smaller pieces and steep them as a tea. The resulting tincture is going to give you a host of health benefits without any of the side effects, and you will be back on your feet and ready to take on the world again in no time.

From mild aches and pains that you feel from your age or activities to the aches and pains that are caused by illness, you can effectively treat them all with essential oils and herbs.

Let me show you exactly what you need to do to rid yourself of the aches and pains you have been facing on a daily basis, and give you your mobility back. No more wasted days feeling poorly, no more skipping things you used to enjoy because you don't want to be sore.

With herbal remedies and essential oils, you are going to get the relief you need without breaking the bank. Guaranteed.

Chapter 2 – Essential Oils and Aromatherapy: Does it Work?

When it comes to using essential oils for your health, you really can't go wrong. These oils have been around for hundreds of years, and possess incredibly healing powers.

An essential oil is a concentrated oil derived from a plant. More often than not, the oils are taken from the fruit or leaves of the plant, but they can also come from the seeds or roots as well.

When it comes to using essential oils for your health, you must choose oils that are pure. Look for the words "therapy grade" and "100% pure" as you shop for your oils, and check to ensure that the oils come in dark bottles.

Essential oils require dark glass bottles to stay potent, so anything found in a light bottle is likely not pure oil.

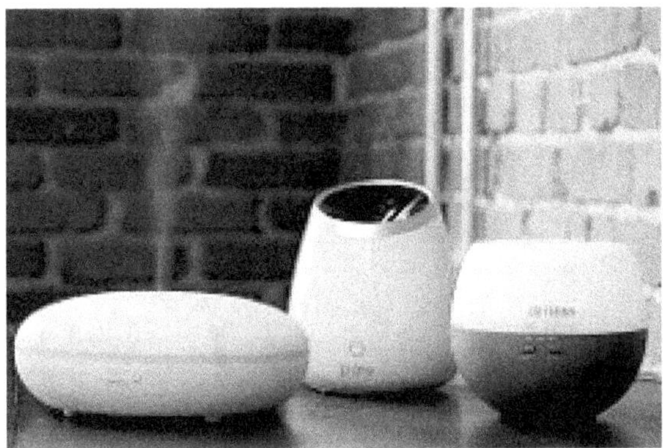

Once you have chosen your oils, you must then choose your diffuser. Diffusers can be purchased online and at a variety of health stores, so you aren't going to have any trouble with obtaining your own. With dozens of styles in a variety of materials available, you are going to have the opportunity to pick just what you want for your décor.

Depending on the size of the diffuser, you can run it continuously for up to 12 hours. The smaller tanks tend to hover around 2 to 4 hours, but you can choose the size you want as you shop around.

How effective is aromatherapy?

In several studies, aromatherapy has proven to be every bit as effective as conventional medicine when it comes to treating a variety of ailments. People who have had trouble focusing report that aromatherapy makes their mind sharper.

It relieves anxiety and headaches, depression and a host of other common ailments. When mixed with a carrier oil and applied directly to the skin, they have proven to be as effective as a host of creams and ointments as well.

Treat stomachaches, joint aches, muscle cramps, and virtually anything else you want to treat through these oils, and forget the conventional medication.

Can you overdose on essential oils?

It is debatable whether these oils are safe to ingest, so I recommend you do not. If you use them in your diffuser as the diffuser is intended to be used, then there is no possible way to overdose on the oils.

However, if you are applying the oils directly to your skin, you must blend them with a carrier oil as a high concentration can cause skin irritation and even burns. Keep the oils out of reach of children at all times, and always personally apply the oils if you are using them on a child.

All in all, you are going to fall in love with essential oils and aromatherapy. Once you discover not only how easy they are to make but how effective they are in treating illness, you'll never want to go back.

Here are the recipes to get you started on your path to natural success. Whip up a blend and fill your diffuser, and experience the magic today.

Chapter 3 – Essential Oil Recipes for Natural Relief

Now is the time to put this knowledge to use! Here are the essential oils recipes you need to find relief for sore and aching joints, aches and pains due to illness, and relief for mental pain and anxiety.

You can use a diffuser for many of the blends, allowing the goodness to fill the air. However, for direct application, combine each blend with a carrier oil and massage externally onto the affected area.

Do not ingest the oils.

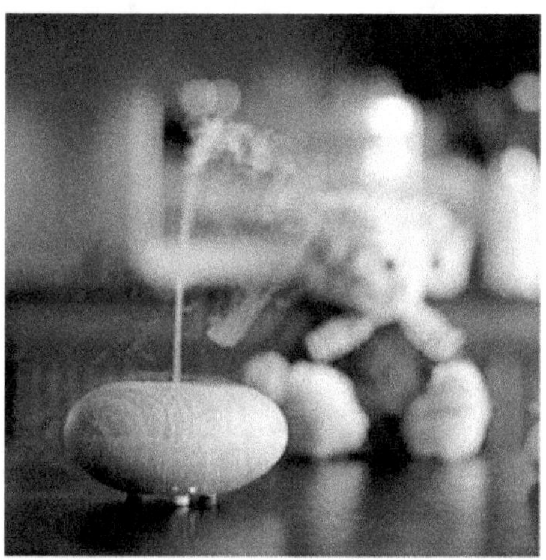

The Good Stuff
What you will need:

10 drops lavender

10 drops chamomile

5 drops rose

Directions:

If you are using a diffuser, you will combine the essential oils in a jar and shake well, then you will transfer the oils from the jar to the diffuser, filling it with water according to your diffuser's directions.

Plug in diffuser and let the aromatherapy fill the air, giving you the relief you need.

For direct application, combine the oils in a jar and shake well, then combine them with 2 tablespoons fractionated coconut oil and massage into the affected area.

Repeat morning and night, or as needed.

Young Again

What you will need:

10 drops myrrh

10 drops vanilla essential oil

Directions:

If you are using a diffuser, you will combine the essential oils in a jar and shake well, then you will transfer the oils from the jar to the diffuser, filling it with water according to your diffuser's directions.

Plug in diffuser and let the aromatherapy fill the air, giving you the relief you need.

For direct application, combine the oils in a jar and shake well, then combine them with 2 tablespoons fractionated coconut oil and massage into the affected area.

Repeat morning and night, or as needed.

Instant Burn Relief
What you will need:

10 drops myrrh

8 drops eucalyptus

Directions:

For direct application, combine the oils in a jar and shake well, then combine them with 2 tablespoons fractionated coconut oil and massage into the affected area.

Repeat morning and night, or as needed.

Clear Focus
What you will need:

10 drops peppermint

8 drops spearmint

8 drops eucalyptus

Directions:

If you are using a diffuser, you will combine the essential oils in a jar and shake well, then you will transfer the oils from the jar to the diffuser, filling it with water according to your diffuser's directions.

Plug in diffuser and let the aromatherapy fill the air, giving you the relief you need.

For direct application, combine the oils in a jar and shake well, then combine them with 2 tablespoons fractionated coconut oil and massage into the affected area.

Repeat morning and night, or as needed.

Worry Away

What you will need:

10 drops peppermint

8 drops lavender

8 drops lemon

Directions:

If you are using a diffuser, you will combine the essential oils in a jar and shake well, then you will transfer the oils from the jar to the diffuser, filling it with water according to your diffuser's directions.

Plug in diffuser and let the aromatherapy fill the air, giving you the relief you need.

For direct application, combine the oils in a jar and shake well, then combine them with 2 tablespoons fractionated coconut oil and massage into the affected area.

Repeat morning and night, or as needed.

Healthy Joint Juice

What you will need:

8 drops cinnamon

9 drops frankincense

9 drops myrrh

Directions:

For direct application, combine the oils in a jar and shake well, then combine them with 2 tablespoons fractionated coconut oil and massage into the affected area.

Repeat morning and night, or as needed.

Headache Healer

What you will need:

10 drops peppermint

8 drops geranium

8 drops ginger

Directions:

If you are using a diffuser, you will combine the essential oils in a jar and shake well, then you will transfer the oils from the jar to the diffuser, filling it with water according to your diffuser's directions.

Plug in diffuser and let the aromatherapy fill the air, giving you the relief you need.

For direct application, combine the oils in a jar and shake well, then combine them with 2 tablespoons fractionated coconut oil and massage into the affected area.

Repeat morning and night, or as needed.

Back Booster

What you will need:

12 drops frankincense

8 drops blood orange

8 drops lemon

Directions:

For direct application, combine the oils in a jar and shake well, then combine them with 2 tablespoons fractionated coconut oil and massage into the affected area.

Repeat morning and night, or as needed.

Muscle Magic

What you will need:

12 drops grapefruit

8 drops cinnamon

8 drops lemon

Directions:

For direct application, combine the oils in a jar and shake well, then combine them with 2 tablespoons fractionated coconut oil and massage into the affected area.

Repeat morning and night, or as needed.

Happy Days
What you will need:

11 drops chamomile

8 drops lavender

8 drops lemon

Directions:

If you are using a diffuser, you will combine the essential oils in a jar and shake well, then you will transfer the oils from the jar to the diffuser, filling it with water according to your diffuser's directions.

Plug in diffuser and let the aromatherapy fill the air, giving you the relief you need.

For direct application, combine the oils in a jar and shake well, then combine them with 2 tablespoons fractionated coconut oil and massage into the affected area.

Repeat morning and night, or as needed.

Move Freely
What you will need:

12 drops myrrh

8 drops goldenseal

8 drops sandalwood

Directions:

If you are using a diffuser, you will combine the essential oils in a jar and shake well, then you will transfer the oils from the jar to the diffuser, filling it with water according to your diffuser's directions.

Plug in diffuser and let the aromatherapy fill the air, giving you the relief you need.

For direct application, combine the oils in a jar and shake well, then combine them with 2 tablespoons fractionated coconut oil and massage into the affected area.

Repeat morning and night, or as needed.

Tummy Ache Tamer
What you will need:

12 drops peppermint

12 drops ginger

4 drops eucalyptus

Directions:

For direct application, combine the oils in a jar and shake well, then combine them with 2 tablespoons fractionated coconut oil and massage into the affected area.

Repeat morning and night, or as needed.

Stiffness Be Gone

What you will need:

12 drops geranium

8 drops tea tree oil

8 drops myrrh

Directions:

For direct application, combine the oils in a jar and shake well, then combine them with 2 tablespoons fractionated coconut oil and massage into the affected area.

Repeat morning and night, or as needed.

Jump for Joy

What you will need:

10 drops grapefruit

8 drops tea tree oil

5 drops fir needle

Directions:

If you are using a diffuser, you will combine the essential oils in a jar and shake well, then you will transfer the oils from the jar to the diffuser, filling it with water according to your diffuser's directions.

Plug in diffuser and let the aromatherapy fill the air, giving you the relief you need.

For direct application, combine the oils in a jar and shake well, then combine them with 2 tablespoons fractionated coconut oil and massage into the affected area.

Repeat morning and night, or as needed.

Totally Moveable Blend

What you will need:

10 drops cinnamon

8 drops basil

8 drops patchouli

Directions:

If you are using a diffuser, you will combine the essential oils in a jar and shake well, then you will transfer the oils from the jar to the diffuser, filling it with water according to your diffuser's directions.

Plug in diffuser and let the aromatherapy fill the air, giving you the relief you need.

For direct application, combine the oils in a jar and shake well, then combine them with 2 tablespoons fractionated coconut oil and massage into the affected area.

Repeat morning and night, or as needed.

The Athlete's Choice

What you will need:

10 drops rose

8 drops rosewood

8 drops peppermint

Directions:

If you are using a diffuser, you will combine the essential oils in a jar and shake well, then you will transfer the oils from the jar to the diffuser, filling it with water according to your diffuser's directions.

Plug in diffuser and let the aromatherapy fill the air, giving you the relief you need.

For direct application, combine the oils in a jar and shake well, then combine them with 2 tablespoons fractionated coconut oil and massage into the affected area.

Repeat morning and night, or as needed.

Flu Fighter
What you will need:

10 drops cinnamon

10 drops ginger

8 drops blood orange

Directions:

If you are using a diffuser, you will combine the essential oils in a jar and shake well, then you will transfer the oils from the jar to the diffuser, filling it with water according to your diffuser's directions.

Plug in diffuser and let the aromatherapy fill the air, giving you the relief you need.

For direct application, combine the oils in a jar and shake well, then combine them with 2 tablespoons fractionated coconut oil and massage into the affected area.

Repeat morning and night, or as needed.

Sore Throat Soother
What you will need:

12 drops cinnamon

12 drops peppermint

Directions:

If you are using a diffuser, you will combine the essential oils in a jar and shake well, then you will transfer the oils from the jar to the diffuser, filling it with water according to your diffuser's directions.

Plug in diffuser and let the aromatherapy fill the air, giving you the relief you need.

For direct application, combine the oils in a jar and shake well, then combine them with 2 tablespoons fractionated coconut oil and massage externally into the affected area.

Repeat morning and night, or as needed.

Good Mood Melody
What you will need:

10 drops lavender

10 drops myrrh

10 drops chamomile

Directions:

If you are using a diffuser, you will combine the essential oils in a jar and shake well, then you will transfer the oils from the jar to the diffuser, filling it with water according to your diffuser's directions.

Plug in diffuser and let the aromatherapy fill the air, giving you the relief you need.

For direct application, combine the oils in a jar and shake well, then combine them with 2 tablespoons fractionated coconut oil and massage into the affected area.

Repeat morning and night, or as needed.

Background Bliss
What you will need:

10 drops sunflower essential oil

10 drops vanilla essential oil

8 drops geranium oil

Directions:

If you are using a diffuser, you will combine the essential oils in a jar and shake well, then you will transfer the oils from the jar to the diffuser, filling it with water according to your diffuser's directions.

Plug in diffuser and let the aromatherapy fill the air, giving you the relief you need.

For direct application, combine the oils in a jar and shake well, then combine them with 2 tablespoons fractionated coconut oil and massage into the affected area.

Repeat morning and night, or as needed.

Chapter 4 – Herbal Teas and Tonics

I highly recommend you get a diffuser, and that you practice aromatherapy often, however, in addition to the aromatherapy, you may need that extra boost from time to time, and that's best in the form of a tea or tonic.

Herbal remedies have held their own for as long as mankind has existed, and in spite of the modern medicine, they continue to maintain their elevated stance.

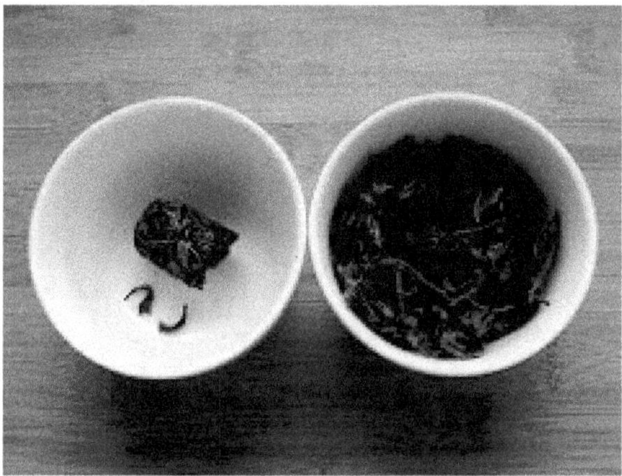

Try these blends for your ailments, and start feeling better in no time at all – without any of the side effects:

Get up and Go
What you will need:

2 teaspoons chopped ginger root

1 teaspoon chopped turmeric root

2 teaspoons black tea leaves

Honey

Directions:

Make sure all leaves and ingredients are broken into small bits and pieces. Wrap these in tea paper or place them in a tea ball.

Fill a mug with hot water, then place your tea blend in this mug. Allow to steep for at least 5 minutes before you sip on it.

I recommend you leave the ball in the water for a total of 15 minutes before you take it out. Enjoy a glass of tea in the morning and late afternoon, or whenever you need an extra boost.

Stomach Soother
What you will need:

2 teaspoons peppermint leaves

2 teaspoons black tea leaves

1 teaspoon chopped ginger root

Honey

Directions:

Make sure all leaves and ingredients are broken into small bits and pieces. Wrap these in tea paper or place them in a tea ball.

Fill a mug with hot water, then place your tea blend in this mug. Allow to steep for at least 5 minutes before you sip on it.

I recommend you leave the ball in the water for a total of 15 minutes before you take it out. Enjoy a glass of tea in the morning and late afternoon, or whenever you need an extra boost.

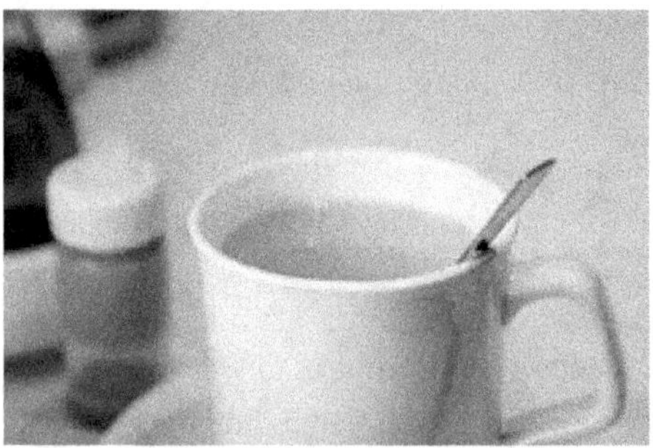

Sore Throat Banisher
What you will need:

1 teaspoon licorice root

2 teaspoons black tea leaves

¼ teaspoon cayenne pepper

Honey

Directions:

Make sure all leaves and ingredients are broken into small bits and pieces. Wrap these in tea paper or place them in a tea ball.

Fill a mug with hot water, then place your tea blend in this mug. Allow to steep for at least 5 minutes before you sip on it.

I recommend you leave the ball in the water for a total of 15 minutes before you take it out. Enjoy a glass of tea in the morning and late afternoon, or whenever you need an extra boost.

Cold and Flu Super Hero

What you will need:

1 tablespoon dried organic lemon peel

2 teaspoons black tea leaves

1 teaspoon ground marshmallow leaves

1 teaspoon mint leaves

Directions:

Make sure all leaves and ingredients are broken into small bits and pieces. Wrap these in tea paper or place them in a tea ball.

Fill a mug with hot water, then place your tea blend in this mug. Allow to steep for at least 5 minutes before you sip on it.

I recommend you leave the ball in the water for a total of 15 minutes before you take it out. Enjoy a glass of tea in the morning and late afternoon, or whenever you need an extra boost.

Achy Breaky Blend

What you will need:

1 teaspoon St. John's Wort leaves

2 teaspoons ginseng leaves

2 teaspoons black tea leaves

Honey

Directions:

Make sure all leaves and ingredients are broken into small bits and pieces. Wrap these in tea paper or place them in a tea ball.

Fill a mug with hot water, then place your tea blend in this mug. Allow to steep for at least 5 minutes before you sip on it.

I recommend you leave the ball in the water for a total of 15 minutes before you take it out. Enjoy a glass of tea in the morning and late afternoon, or whenever you need an extra boost.

Best for the Rest Tea Tonic
What you will need:

1 teaspoon valerian root

2 teaspoons black tea leaves

1 teaspoon chamomile leaves

Honey

1 tablespoon apple cider vinegar

Directions:

Make sure all leaves and ingredients are broken into small bits and pieces. Wrap these in tea paper or place them in a tea ball.

Fill a mug with hot water, and add the vinegar, then place your tea blend in this mug. Allow to steep for at least 5 minutes before you sip on it.

I recommend you leave the ball in the water for a total of 15 minutes before you take it out. Enjoy a glass of tea in the morning and late afternoon, or whenever you need an extra boost.

Apple Might
What you will need:

1 tablespoon apple cider vinegar

1 teaspoon cinnamon bark

1 tablespoon dehydrated apples

1 teaspoon ground ginger

2 teaspoons black tea leaves

Honey

Directions:

Make sure all leaves and ingredients are broken into small bits and pieces. Wrap these in tea paper or place them in a tea ball.

Fill a mug with hot water, then place your tea blend in this mug. Allow to steep for at least 5 minutes before you sip on it.

I recommend you leave the ball in the water for a total of 15 minutes before you take it out. Enjoy a glass of tea in the morning and late afternoon, or whenever you need an extra boost.

Peach and Longevity
What you will need:

2 teaspoons ground peach pit

1 teaspoon ginger root

2 teaspoons black tea leaves

Honey

Directions:

Make sure all leaves and ingredients are broken into small bits and pieces. Wrap these in tea paper or place them in a tea ball.

Fill a mug with hot water, then place your tea blend in this mug. Allow to steep for at least 5 minutes before you sip on it.

I recommend you leave the ball in the water for a total of 15 minutes before you take it out. Enjoy a glass of tea in the morning and late afternoon, or whenever you need an extra boost.

His and Hers
What you will need:

2 teaspoons ground rosehips

1 teaspoon raspberry leaves

2 teaspoons black tea leaves

Honey

Directions:

Make sure all leaves and ingredients are broken into small bits and pieces. Wrap these in tea paper or place them in a tea ball.

Fill a mug with hot water, then place your tea blend in this mug. Allow to steep for at least 5 minutes before you sip on it.

I recommend you leave the ball in the water for a total of 15 minutes before you take it out. Enjoy a glass of tea in the morning and late afternoon, or whenever you need an extra boost.

Everything's All Right

What you will need:

2 teaspoons ginseng leaves

2 teaspoons raspberry leaves

1 teaspoon ginger root

2 teaspoons black tea leaves

1 teaspoon turmeric root

Honey

Directions:

Make sure all leaves and ingredients are broken into small bits and pieces. Wrap these in tea paper or place them in a tea ball.

Fill a mug with hot water, then place your tea blend in this mug. Allow to steep for at least 5 minutes before you sip on it.

I recommend you leave the ball in the water for a total of 15 minutes before you take it out. Enjoy a glass of tea in the morning and late afternoon, or whenever you need an extra boost.

Conclusion

There you have it, everything you need to know about aromatherapy, essential oils, and how to use herbs for home remedies and pain relief. I hope this book inspires you to turn to the natural remedies when you are searching for healing rather than the conventional medication.

Though there are certainly times when it is best to go with the conventional, you don't want to be so wrapped up in conventional remedies that you forget to treat your body as it was meant to be treated – naturally.

With this book, I want you to break out of the conventional line of thinking, and start embracing natural remedies for your aches and pains. You never know when you are going to run into side effects that leave you in a worse condition than you were in in the first place, and when you use essential oils and herbal remedies, you never have to worry about such things.

My goal is to educate and inspire, giving you the solutions you need to get the results you want. Say goodbye to pain and aches, and not being able to move like you used to. Whether you are an athlete who is tired of always feeling sore after workouts, or if you are someone who just isn't as young as you used to be, you will find what you need in these remedies.

And don't stop here. With this book, you are going to learn the tools you need to jump start an actively natural life, meaning you can always turn to natural remedies regardless of the pain you are dealing with.

Don't reach for that bottle of pills filled with side effects, instead, reach for a warm cup of soothing tea while your diffuser fills the air with warmth in the background. This is going to relax you, give you the results you want, and show you how you can use natural remedies for your natural ailments.

Let this book be your guide in the natural world, and jump start and all natural pain and body ache solution that will leave you feeling like you are on top of the world once again.

There's no end to the ways you can indulge in natural remedies, and the better you get at it, the easier it's going to be to add to your skills. Dive into the world of the all natural, and leave pain and body aches in the dust.

Good luck!

FREE Bonus Reminder

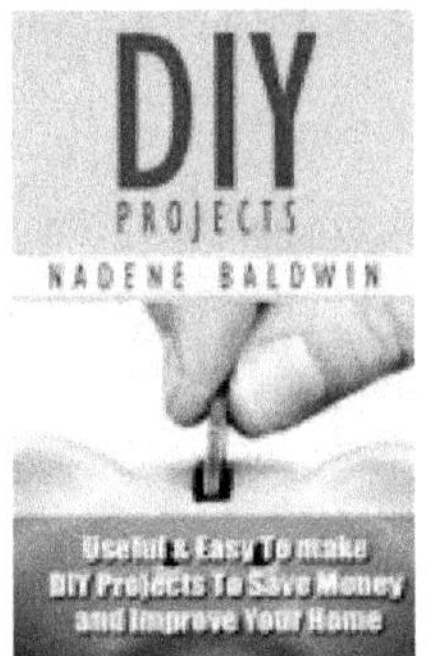

If you have not grabbed it yet, please go ahead and download your special bonus report *"DIY Projects. 13 Useful & Easy To Make DIY Projects To Save Money & Improve Your Home!"*

Simply Click the Button Below

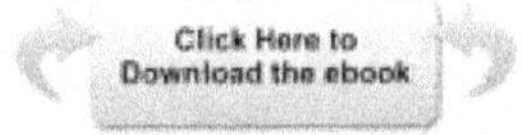

OR **Go to This Page**

http://diyhomecraft.com/free

BONUS #2: More Free & Discounted Books or Products

Do you want to receive more Free/Discounted Books or Products?

We have a mailing list where we send out our new Books or Products when they go free or with a discount on Amazon. Click on the link below to sign up for Free & Discount Book & Product Promotions.

=> Sign Up for Free & Discount Book & Product Promotions <=

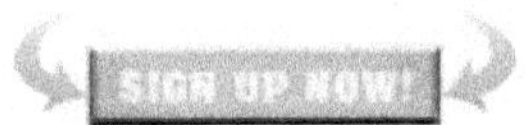

OR Go to this URL

http://zbit.ly/1WBb1Ek